Elements of Medical Jurisprudence

46169.

Printed by Smith & Davy,
17, Queen Street, Seven Dials.

PREFACE.

THE foundation of this little Work is taken from a Publication made at Geneva in the year 1767, called, 'Joh. Fred. Faselii Elementa Medicinæ Forensis.' This was a class-book of a learned Professor; but I imagined such a form, and boundless divisions which he has adopted, would appear tedious to an English reader, who generally admires works more in detail. I have therefore admitted only the materials of that publication, and have digested them into regular chapters, in which I have endeavoured, as much as possible, to follow the order of nature, beginning with births, and ending with the dissolution of our frame.

By altering the form too, I have not been obliged to adhere strictly to the text, but have varied from it very

B   considerably;

considerably; and some chapters I have entirely added, as that upon Madness, &c. whilst others I have omitted as useless in this country, as particularly one on Tortures, &c. But I hope I have neither added what is tedious, nor omitted what is necessary to be known. As nothing of the kind hath ever been published in this country, I was willing to take the assistance of a learned foreigner, rather than travel a tract unbeaten by myself. I need say nothing concerning the utility of such a Work; it will readily be pointed out to every serious mind. Life and death are objects too important to be sported with in the manner they are sometimes: nor should the valuable connections of our fellow-citizens be ever sacrificed to the ignorance of the faculty, the caprice of a court, or the artifices of revenge and disappointment.

SAMUEL FARR.

Curry-Rivel,
Nov. 22, 1787.

CONTENTS.

B 2

INSTITUTES, &c.

INTRODUCTION.

THERE is a kind of medical knowledge, which is not so much concerned in the cure of diseases, as in the detection of error, and the conviction of guilt. A physician, a surgeon, or a coroner, is often called upon to make a deposition of what he knows concerning some particular transactions in a court of judicature. Such persons then should be well acquainted with the animal œconomy; and with those views of the science, which, in foreign countries, have been dignified with a peculiar name, as the medicine of the courts, legal medicine, or medical jurisprudence.

B 3   This

This knowledge, in its more extensive sense, is divided into two different kinds, in one of which is explained those rules by which a judge may form in a court of judicature, an accurate opinion of the cause which comes before him: in the other, an acquaintance is acquired with the best methods of preserving the health of our fellow citizens. The first part is again divided into three, as the deposition is made in the civil courts, in the criminal courts, or in the ecclesiastical courts. But as the courts of foreign countries are constituted upon different principles from those of this kingdom, I shall not follow the example of our learned professor, in arranging the rules of this business in that division, but shall give them in different chapters, according to the order of Nature, and let the reader apply them as he shall think proper.

How divided.

Judicial causes.

Health of community.

Natural division.

CHAP.

CHAP. I.

OF PREGNANCY.

THERE are so many decisions, both
in civil and criminal courts dependent
upon pregnancy, that an accurate
knowledge of this affection is absolutely necessary to be acquired before
a determination is made. And notwithstanding there may be an appa-
rent indecency in the exposition, yet
truth, property, and perhaps a life,
are not to be sacrificed to a false delicacy, a mistaken modesty, or a love
of ease.

*Many de-
cisions de-
pend on a
knowledge
of it.*

A greater expansion of the abdomen than common, as it creates in a
female the idea of pregnancy, may
depend upon a foetus, or any other
body, filling up the womb, or parts
adjacent. If it be any foreign body,
it is called a mole, or false conception;

*Marks of
pregnan-
cy.*

*Distin-
guished
from other
appearan-
ces.*

Mole what.

B 4

tion; if a fœtus, true pregnancy. This too is of two kinds, ordinary and

Ordinary.

extraordinary. The first, when one or more fœtuses are lodged in the hollow of the womb itself; the latter,

Extraordinary.

when they are deposited in the ovarium, the fallopian tube, or the general cavity of the abdomen. The ovarium is that substance in the female body, which answers to the testicle in that of the male, and is supposed to contain the germen of the future animal. The fallopian tube is a duct which conveys the male semen from the womb to the ovarium, and is supposed to embrace the uterus in the time of conception. It is natural to suppose then, that sometimes the fœtus may be lodged in these bodies, and seek an exit which it can never obtain.

It is not uncommon for women of abandoned characters, or even married women, to conceal and deny their state of pregnancy; and in such cases,

no

no accurate judgment can be formed
till a proper examination be made by
a medical person, and those signs of
true pregnancy be discovered which
are generally acknowledged. These
signs are various, and they may be, Signs.
distinguished into certain, uncertain,
and false.

The certain and most common, Certain.
and which may be taken about the
time when half the gestation is com-
pleated, are :

1st. A swelling of the abdomen, Swelling of abdomen.
which arises from no morbid cause,
which continues to increase so, that it
extends from the lower part even to
the summit, which has a shining appearance, and which is peculiarly
sharpened about the navel. At the
same time a troublesome sensation, peculiar to such a situation, is perceived,
and other signs of pregnancy occur.

2d. The orifice of the womb is Orifice of the womb. altered.
thicker, more spongy, soft, and wi-
B 5 dened;

dened; is shorter, and exhibits neither a conical nor cylindrical figure.

Motion of fœtus.

3d. A motion of the fœtus is perceived in the womb.

Suppression of menses.

4th. There is a suppression of the menstrual flux, when it cannot be accounted for from some evident disease, and when the symptoms which accompany it do not remit, as is the case when it arises from some other cause.

Swelling of breasts.

5th. A swelling and hardness of the breasts, with an inflation of the nipple, and the veins of the breasts assuming a blue colour. The disk round the nipple is of a dusky brown colour, and the little eminences are much enlarged.

Milk in breasts.

6th. A lymph flows from the breast upon pressure, which are streaks of true milk.

Uncertain signs of pregnancy.

The uncertain signs of pregnancy, are frequent vomitings, especially in a morning; a constipation of the belly; an incontinence or suppression of of urine, difficult respiration, irregular appetite, a fondness or aversion to particular kinds of food, head-ach, vertigo, pain of the teeth, yellow spots in the face, the belly growing flat, a descent of the orifice of the womb, enlargement of the veins, swelling of the legs and feet, and pains in the loins, &c.

The false signs of pregnancy have *False signs.* arisen from some superstitious notions which are now exploded, and therefore we shall omit to mention them in this place.

It appears, however, that no accurate judgment can be formed, but *How to form a judgment.* from the certain signs; and a knowledge of these can only be acquired by a minute examination and immediate inspection of the parts. This, upon account of decency, is generally committed to midwives, ignorant persons, who have no knowledge of the animal œconomy, and may easily be deceived.

B 6

ceived. It would be much better then, that this office should be entrusted to the more regular practitioner, who being a person of education, would add the influence of his judgment to his examination, and would not be content with a single enquiry, which may be uncertain, but would frequently repeat it, till he had perfectly ascertained the truth.

Feigned pregnancy.

Women sometimes likewise feign themselves to be pregnant when they are not so. The absence of those

How discovered.

signs before described, would be sufficient to confute them; but, as much artifice is often used upon such occasions, it may be necessary to examine a little further, and here the following

Signs.

signs presents themselves: An improper age, either too tender or too perfect; a preternatural defect of the menses, even in those of a fit age; too great a flow of them; a copious and inveterate fluor albus; various diseases

diseases of the vagina, as the orifice of it being entirely shut, or a junction of its sides, so as not to admit of an entrance; various diseases likewise of the womb, such as schirrus, or fleshy excrescences growing up in it, or its mouth being entirely closed.

CHAP.

CHAP. II.

_____

OF PARTURITION OR CHILD-BIRTH.

Parturition
what.

PARTURITION may be received in several senses. At one time it means the action of bringing a child into the world: at another the child itself, which is received into being.

Ordinary.

When taken in the first sense, it is divided into ordinary and extraordinary. The ordinary is, when the delivery is made in the common and usual manner, or rather by the common passages, notwithstanding any difficulties which may occur in the operation: for this is again divided into natural and preternatural, or arti-

Extraordi-
nary.
Cæsarean
operation.

ficial. The extraordinary delivery is when it is performed by the Cæsarean operation, which is an extraction of
the

the child, by making an incision through the abdominal muscles into the uterus. This is seldom performed upon the living mother, but may be, and is indeed always advisable, should the mother die before she can be delivered, and life is perceived in the child. In this way some great personages, and particularly our Edward VI. is said to have been born. Another method lately proposed in France, and absolutely put in practice upon living subjects, is, by dividing the cartilage which binds together the bones that surround the womb, and thus enlarging the opening. This may likewise be called extraordinary, though the delivery be made by the natural passages; yet the strictness of terms confines it to those labours which are made by passages different from the common.

When the word parturition relates to the child itself, it may denote the time when it is born, the conformation

When parturition relates to the child.

of

of its parts, or the external figure which it presents, the state of its life, and the number which are brought into the world.

Time of birth.

When it relates to the time in which it is born, it may be considered

Perfect.

either as perfect or mature, or immature and imperfect. The former, when gestation has been carried on at least

Imperfect.

nine months: the latter, when it is completed before that time; and in this last case, another division may be

Abortions.

made into abortions, where the delivery is made before the seventh month;

Premature.

and premature births, where the child is born between the seventh and the end of the ninth. To this head also belong too late deliveries.

Signs of immature child.

The signs of an immature child are taken from the following particulars.

Length.

1st. From its length, for if it be not one foot long, we may be nearly certain that it is not completely formed.

2d.

2d. From its weight, which should exceed five pounds. Weight.

3d. From the figure of the head, &c. An incomplete child has a deformed face resembling an old person, with a wide mouth and slender ears like membranes; its eyes are shut; the hair of its head is of a whitish cast; the division between the bones of the skull, called the rhomfoidal suture, gapes wide; the bones themselves are moveable; and the lips of the mouth resemble pieces of bloody flesh. Figure of parts, &c.

4th. From its habit of body, which is for the most part thin and tender, and covered with a short down, and is of a reddish hue, particularly on the extremities and the face. If it be a male, the scrotum is of a round figure, and the testicles are not contained in it. Habit of body.

5th. From its limbs, which are thin and weak, and the nails upon its Limbs.

fingers

fingers are soft, short, not extending beyond the fingers; nay, if it be very small, as of one or two months, the nails are by no means perceptible, either upon the fingers or the toes.

6th. From the conformation or constitution of its bones; for it is evident from experience, that in every month of gestation, there is some alteration in this respect; ex. gr. in a fœtus of five months, the orbits of the eyes are entirely formed into bony sockets; and in one of seven months, the small bones, subservient to the organ of hearing are so perfect, as scarcely to differ from those of a complete child.

Umbilical cord.

7th. From the umbilical cord, which is very slender.

Other circumstances.

8th. From other curious circumstances which attend this little embryo, such as a constant indulgence in sleep, an abstaining from crying, an intolerance of cold, an indisposition to suck,

suck, or to use its limbs, or the muscles of other parts, such as those which are subservient to the evacuation of urine, òr the depositing of the meconium.

The signs by which we distinguish a perfect child are taken, _{Signs of perfect child.}

1st. From its size ; its length being at least one foot six inches. _{Size.}

2d. From its weight, which should be at least six pounds. _{Weight.}

3d. From the formation of its bones, which is known only by experience. But in general, a child can hardly be called complete, all whose bones, and every part are not entirely formed, though age may give some addition to their substance. _{Formation of bones.}

4th. From the umbilical cord, which is thick and firm. _{Umbilical cord.}

5th. From other circumstances, opposite to those in that which was imperfect ; such as that he cries, moves his limbs, opens his eyes, sucks at the
breast,

breast, is not always asleep, can bear cold, has a white skin, can evacuate urine and the fæces, has long nails, and his head covered with hair.

That which relates to the conformation of a child, after it is brought into the world, is distinguished into monstrous, and not monstrous: the former including all deviations from the ordinary figure of man. Monsters are again divided into perfect and imperfect. A perfect monster is that which absolutely differs in all its parts, from the human appearance, as when it resembles any brute animals, as a dog, an ape, &c. An imperfect monster is where only a partial alteration is made in its figure; and this may again differ, according as this partial alteration is made in the head, or other parts; and this as it may be born without a head, or with the head of a beast, &c. Where a monster differs from a complete child, in other parts besides

Monsters what.

Perfect.

Imperfect.

besides the head, it is distinguished
into two sorts, as any parts in general
are affected, or as more particularly
the change is wrought in the genitals
only, and then it is called an herma- Herma-
phrodite.
phrodite, which is likewise perfect or
imperfect.

In an enquiry into the nature of
monsters in general, three objects of
consideration present themselves. 1st.
What is the cause of monsters? 2d.
Whether they are possessed of life?
3d. Whether a perfect monster can be
considered as a human being?

1st. The cause of monsters is vari- Cause of
Monsters.
ous, as depending on such changes in
the constitution of the mother, as can
hardly be accounted for.

Whatever view we take of the Theory of
generati-
on.
theory of generation, whether a ger-
men be formed in the ovarium of the
female, which is only impregnated by
the semen of the male, or whether the
homunculus is contained in that semen,

men, and the female affords a nidus for
its formation; still we see a strong
resemblance to both parents in their
offspring: and accidents, or other
causes, contribute to make an entire
alteration in the form of the fœtus,
and produce monsters. We will not
suppose unnatural connections, or that
any impregnation can arise from that
source; but imagination has a great
power over the body of a female,
especially during gestation; and the
fluid in which the fœtus swims, or the
womb itself may be disordered, so as
to occasion great changes. Neither
need we have recourse to the theory of the ingenious Buffon to explain
how these are brought about; or suppose that every part of the human body has a representation in the fecun-
dating quality of both parents, to form
its construction. The first rudiments or germen of the human body
is not a human creature, if it be even
a living

a living one; it is a foundation only
upon which the human superstructure
is raised. This is evident to anatomical observation. Were a child to be
born of the shape which it presents in
the first stages of pregnancy, it would
be a monster indeed, as great as any
which was ever brought to light. How
easy then is it for disorder to prevent
the exertion of that plastic force,
which is necessary to form a complete
animal.

2d. Monsters may live, but it de- Whether
pends on what parts are affected, how monsters can live.
long life shall be continued to them.
Where the monstrous parts are confined to the extremities, or even to
those places which distinguish hermaphrodites, we find from experience,
that the vital powers are strong and
vigorous; and were it not that such
beings often fly from society, lead
sedentary lives, and are deprived of
some wholesome exercises to the human

man constitution, life might be enjoyed by them, and to as great an extent as by any other persons. .

Are there perfect monsters? · 3d. With regard to perfect monsters, most of the authorities which assert that any thing of that kind can exist, seem to be of no credit. But should any ever appear, we should consider that it is not form or shape, but reason and intelligence, which distinguish human creatures from brute animals.

Hermaphrodites what. ·We are next to consider the nature of hermaphrodites; and as these are living beings, and sometimes capable of all the functions of society, such distinctions ought to be made relating to them, as will place their situation in the most proper light, and the most favourable to their happiness. They are great objects of our pity and complacency; for they are not only deprived of the common pleasures of mankind, but are subject to disorders which

which are painful, uncomfortable, and
inconvenient. A perfect hermaphro- *Perfect.*
dite, or a being partaking of the dis-
tinguishing marks of both sexes, with
a power of enjoyment from each, is
not believed by any one ever to have
existed. Imperfect hermaphrodites, *Imperfect.*
or monsters, whose organs of generation are affected, are frequently pre-
sented to us. They may be divided,
according to the sexes, into what are
called androgynus, and androgyna.
The first is the male, who has in ge- *Androgy-*
neral his own organs tolerably per- *nus.*
fect, but has some division in the flesh
above, below, on, or in the scrotum,
which puts on the appearance of the
female pudendum. The penis likewise may be so obliterated, as to give
no external appearance of the male;
but the beard, and the constitution of
his body, confirm him to be of that
sex. The androgyna is a woman, *Androgy-*
who has the parts of generation nearly *na.*

like another, but at the same time the clitoris grows to a great size, and gives the form of the male penis. This is a very inconvenient disorder, as she is sometimes deprived of the pleasures peculiar to her sex, and suffers much from disorders of the part. From her breasts, and the deficiency of beard however, she is distinguished from the male; though it frequently and unfortunately happens, that such women are more subject than others to robust and masculine constitutions. It is evident that the sexes here are as completely marked as in other persons, and to all legal intents and purposes, they are man and woman.

Some important enquiries may arise upon this subject. As 1st. How far they are to be considered as impotent. This is, I believe, generally the case, but not always, and must depend upon proof. 2d. Whether they should be permitted to marry? This depends upon

Herma-
phrodites,
how far
impotent.

Should
they mar-
ry?

upon the former, but must, I should think, be left to their own choice. 3d. Whether change of the sexes might be allowed? This is certainly contradicted in the terms, and will admit of no dispute.

May they change sex?

With regard to the state of life of a child, the following question requires to be decided: At what time may a foetus be supposed to begin to live? To answer this, we must consider, that conception is made in the ovarium of a female after coition with a male, when the subtile aura of the semen hath so far penetrated into the germen, which may be supposed to contain the outline of the future man, as to produce a turgescence and motion of its circulating humours. At this time, it may be said, that life begins, *i. e.* immediately after conception. Hence those seem to err: 1st. Who would persuade us, that the foetus acquires life when it is so particularly active,

When does a foetus begin to live?

What is conception?

that

that the mother becomes sensible of its motions. 2d. Those who think that life does not begin till the seventh or fourteenth day, or even till a month after conception. And 3d. Those who suppose that a fœtus, as long as it continues in the womb, where it does not breathe, cannot be called a living animal. The whole depends on our ideas of life and animation, and the act of generation to create it. If generation be the cause of animating the rudiments of the future being, and if that animation be construed to be understood by what is meant by life, then it must certainly begin immediately after conception; and nothing but the arbitrary forms of human institutions can make it otherwise.

On this occasion we may enquire, what part of the human body is the seat of animation, or the soul! To which we answer, that evidently it resides most conspicuously in the brain, because

Seat of the soul.

because that substance being hurt, all
the faculties of the soul become disordered; and because all the nerves of
the body, which are the great instruments of action, are derived from it as
a fountain. But it cannot be supposed that the whole of the brain is
the immediate seat of the soul; it is
probably confined to what is called the
sensorium commune, or a small part
from whence the nerves, destined to
sense and voluntary motions, draw
their origin; as they do likewise from
an appendix to it, called the medulla
oblongata.

The next thing to be considered is,
what kind of children, when born into
the world, are to be deemed endued
with life, or have a prospect of living;
for a fœtus cannot live out of the
womb of its mother!

What children have the power of life.

1st. Then, no abortion can be
said to be endued with life, for if there
be some signs of life when it is brought

No abortion.

c 3   into

into the world, it cannot continue to live, for it can neither take the aliment which is necessary to its sustenance, nor, if it could take it, can it change such gross food into its tender nature. Some authors have asserted, that children of five and six months have lived ; but this is probably a mistake, it being generally agreed, that infants so young cannot sustain the inclemencies to which they must be subject.

Children of seven months.

2d. Children of seven months, or one hundred and eighty-two days after marriage, may live, though generally they are puny, and continue but a short time on earth.

Children above seven months.

3d. All children above seven months are supposed to be endued with vital principles, and of consequence are allowed the privilege of life.

The next subject of consideration, is that of twins, supposititious births, and superfœtation.

The

The right of primogeniture must be determined in natural births, by that which was first born into the world, and which must be decided by the by-standers. If the delivery, however, be made by a passage effected by art, the choice depending on the will of the surgeon, no proper determination can possibly be made.

Twins how considered.

In the affair of supposititious births, two questions occur, according as the birth is performed or not. In the former case, a physician may judge, 1st. From those signs in the mother, which distinguish her having been delivered of a child. 2d. From those signs which refer to her incapacity of conception. 3d. From signs of impotency in the father. 4th. From the umbilical cord in the child not appearing as of one just delivered. Some persons look upon the dissimilitude to the parents to be a sign, but this must be very fallacious. Where the

Supposititious births.

Signs to judge by.

c 4   supposititious

suppositious birth depends on the present state of pregnancy, either the proper signs must be examined, or we must wait the event, should those signs deceive us.

The impregnation of a woman already pregnant, is called a superfœtation. This is either true or false; the former is, when it happens in the womb itself; the latter, when one fœtus is deposited in the womb, the other in the ovarium, the fallopian tube, or the cavity of the abdomen.

Superfœtation.

The following requisites are necessary to a superfœtation. 1st. The pregnant woman ought to bear two children, each of a distinct age. 2d. The delivery of these children should be at different times, at a considerable distance from each other. 3d. The woman must be pregnant, and a nurse at the same time.

Requisites.

There have been many doubts about the reality of this superfœtation, but

but there is no disputing of facts, for which see Gravel on Superfœtation, Eisenman's Anatomical Tables, and the Leipsic Memoirs, 1725.

How this superfœtation is accomplished, is a matter of enquiry, and depends in a great measure on the constitution, or rather the formation of the womb of the mother.

The last thing to be considered under this head of parturition, is the legitimacy or illegality of births; and this is divided into the time when a child is born after conception, and the conformation of its body. With respect to time, physically considered, (for laws may be as arbitrary as they please in this respect) all abortions, too early births, children of nine months, and those who are late born, even to ten months, may be considered as legitimate in old marriages. Illegitimate with respect to the time of birth, are all perfect and mature chil-

c 5   dren,

Legitimacy.

Divided from time.

dren, who are born in the sixth or seventh month after the celebration of marriage; and all late births, when extended to the eleventh, twelfth, or thirteenth month, especially if the husband died of a chronic or lingering disease.

Causes of delay in delivery. There are many causes alleged to occasion a delay or prolongation of delivery, such as great care and anxiety; some severe diseases, as violent hœmorrhages, a phthisical disposition, &c. but these, one should imagine, would rather hasten than retard such a circumstance. Experience is the only guide we can follow in such cases, and, for the sake of humanity, the longest time that can be fairly proved, should be the standard to which we should refer.

Legitimacy from form. With respect to the conformation of the body, all children may be considered legitimate, who are born at or after seven months; but all abortions

are

are illegitimate. Monsters, likewise
are not to be excluded for any trifling
alterations ; but where all appearances
of human nature are obliterated, it
would be wrong to take advantage of
such a birth.

CHAP.

CHAP. III.

ON DIVORCES.

Grounds of divorce. IT is generally allowed, that various disorders may constitute natural grounds for a divorce between two married persons; and notwithstanding the laws of particular countries are generally founded on local customs, and do not always refer to the natural reasons; yet, as no other concern the medical person, and as they are proper to be known, no further apology is necessary for their insertion in this place.

Defects in constitution. Those disorders, or rather as they may be called defects of the human constitution, which seem to constitute the natural reasons for a divorce, are such as are an absolute impediment to the procreation of children. They

They are of two kinds, according as
they have for their subject the organs
of generation or not. The former
may be divided into impotence in
men, and sterility in women, which is
either absolute or *continual,* or such as
eludes all human art to remove.

Absolute impotence in men takes Impotence
place,

1st. When they are eunuchs, or Eunuchs.
are deprived of both testicles, which
being receptacles of the semen, without them no generation can be performed.

2d. When they are spadones, or Spadones.
such as have the nerves or muscles
leading to the parts of generation
bruised, so as to deprive them of all
perception of the venereal appetite.

3d. When the penis is too short, Short pe-
being amputated for disease.   nis.

4th. When the penis is perforated Penis per-
in such a manner that the semen can- forated.
not be thrown out with sufficient force.

This

This rule is to be admitted, with some limitation, as the theory of generation is not sufficiently established to determine with accuracy this point.

Schirrous testicles.

5th. When both testicles are become schirrous, so as not to be capable of a cure.

Semen watery.

6th. When the semen is too watery, and will not admit of amendment. This too being a disease that admits of a cure, should not determine absolutely.

Penis thick.

7th. When the penis is too thick, This is likewise only relative.

Phymosis.

8th. When the preputium is so constructed or fastened to the glans penis, as not to admit of relief by a surgical operation. This disease is called capistration.

Schirrous vesiculæ seminales.

9th. When the vesiculæ seminales are become schirrous.

Diseases grounds for divorce.

Those disorders, which are an impediment to the procreation of children, and which are not derived from the

the organs of generation, are such as
are of a highly contagious nature, or
create an unconquerable aversion; such
as the lues venerea, melancholy, epilepsy, scurvy, scrophula, and a highly
foetid and disagreeable breath. But it
is to be hoped, for the honour of physic, and the benefit of humanity, that
such diseases will meet with their proper cure : and indeed in all the cases
here mentioned, as the happiness of
individuals is so much concerned, and
the public good on the other hand so
much to be studied, it is necessary
that the observations be made with the
greatest care, and that the maturest
judgment of the physician be exercised with discretion.

Absolute sterility in a woman, so Sterility.
as to unfit her for matrimonial duties,
are :

1st. When the parts destined to Parts imperforate.
generation are so imperforate as not to
admit

admit of any relief without incurring great danger of life.

Fluor albus. 2d. When she is so grievously afflicted with the fluor albus, vulgarly called the whites, as not to admit of any cure. Much care and attention are here however requisite, and many medicines are to be tried before an absolute judgment be made: nay, I should think much experience must be admitted, and the husband likewise be examined carefully with regard to his own abilities.

Vagina strait. 3d. When the vagina is too strait and narrow, upon account of schirrous tumours, or of any other kind which it is impossible to remove.

Orifice of womb closed. 4th. When the orifice into the uterus is entirely closed. This will be known not only by the touch, but by the retention of the menstrual flux, which in time will force a passage, or from the dreadful symptoms it induces, require the hand of the surgeon to to procure it. This can hardly be called therefore an absolute impediment.

5th. When there is an ulcer in the uterus, or the passages to it, which sometimes is of so corroding a nature, as to penetrate the rectum and bladder of urine. There are many other causes of sterility, which are derived from injuries or obstructions in the internal parts destined to generation. But here all is darkness, and it would be cruel to determine by any other, than what are quite evident upon inspection and accurate examination of the parts.

Ulcer of womb.

Internal parts diseased.

Before this subject be dismissed, it may be necessary to mention some other circumstances, which, although they may not render either sex absolutely impotent, yet may be considered as defects, and some hindrance to the generative powers, but by no means constitute reasons for a divorce: ignorant

Defects in generation.

norant persons may consider them as such; this error is therefore to be guarded against.

Those which occur in the male sex are, where they are,

Monor-
chides.
1st. Monorchides, or such as have only one testicle. These are by no means incapacitated, as the secretion only is made in that organ from which it is carried to the vesiculæ seminales, and there deposited for use. So that one testicle is as efficacious as two, and the secretion is always proportioned to the evacuation.

Trior-
chides.
2d. Triorchides, or those who have three testicles.

Spadones.
3d. Spadones, where one testicle only is bruised.

Androgy-
ni.
4th. Androgyni, for which see the account of hermaphrodites in the last chapter.

Circumci-
sion.
5th. Those who are circumcised. This is an advantage rather than a hindrance.

6th.

6th. Those who have remedied this defect by art.

Paraphimosis cured.

7th. Chrysporchides, or those whose testicles do not lie in the scrotum, but in the abdomen, or in the groin.

Chrysporchides.

8th. Those who labour under a phimosis, which is a disorder where the præputium is brought over the glans penis, and cannot be retracted but by art.

Phymosis.

9th. Those who have the præputium buttoned over the glans.

Præputium buttoned.

10th. Those whose penis is longer or shorter than natural, unless in very great extremes.

Long and short penis.

Women cannot be said to be incapacitated totally:

Defects in women.

1st. When they have a falling down of the womb; for this may be only temporary, and may be remedied by art.

Prolapsus.

2d. When they have too large a clitoris, or nymphæ.

Large clitoris.

. 3d. When they are androgynæ, or hermaphrodites from other causes.

Androgynæ.

4th.

Parts large.

4th. When they have the pudendum too large and wide.

Flow of menses.

5th. When they have an irregular flow of the menses.

Rupture of perinæum.

6th. When they have suffered in delivery a rupture of the *perinæum,* or the space between the fundament and pudendum.

CHAP.

CHAP. IV.

ON RAPES.

In the consideration of rapes, three objects of attention present themselves.

1st. Whether a rape, strictly so called, be possible? Objects of attention.

2d. Whether a woman, upon a rape being committed, can become pregnant?

3d. What are the signs of a rape being perpetrated?

1st. In answer to the first question, whether a rape be possible, meaning Is a rape possible? upon a grown person, it may be necessary to divide it into two parts, as it is distinguished into the attempt and the consummation of a rape. The Attempt. attempt under which is to be understood a great force exercised over a woman to violate her chastity, but
where

where a compleat coition is prevented, may be possible. But the consummation of a rape, by which is meant a compleat, full, and entire coition, which is made without any consent or permission of the woman, seems to be impossible, unless some very extraordinary circumstances occur: for a woman always possesses sufficient power, by drawing back her limbs, and by the force of her hands, to prevent the insertion of the penis into her body, whilst she can keep her resolution entire. Besides, it is evident that a lesser resistance can prevail against the motion of any body which acts against the weight; and that is the case here: the penis, in attempting an immission into the vagina, moves a body against the weight.

Consummation.

2d. With respect to the next question, whether a woman, upon whom a rape hath been committed, can become pregnant? It may be necessary

Does pregnancy follow a rape?

cessary to enquire how far her lust was excited, or if she experienced any enjoyment. For without an excitation of lust, or the enjoyment of pleasure in the venereal act, no conception can probably take place. So that if an absolute rape were to be perpetrated, it is not likely she would become pregnant.

3d. The signs of a rape having been perpetrated, or rather attempted, are taken from the evacuation of blood from the injured parts, and great swelling and inflammation. But as these may be induced by other means, or are not inconsistent with consent having been obtained, they can only be considered as corroborating, but not as certain proofs.

As rapes however are sometimes committed upon young children, who may have the signs of their virginity obliterated by them, it may be necessary to consider what are those signs, and

and what are the marks of their being Signs of virginity. destroyed. The signs of virginity then may be allowed to be the following.

1st. The lips of the pudendum are more prominent, and close together.

2d. The nymphæ are small, endued with a light rose colour, and do not extend out of their place.

3d. The prepuce of the clitoris is small, and does not cover the glans.

4. The orifice of the urethra, or urinary passage, is entirely covered.

5th. The wrinkles of the vagina are considerable, and raised above the surface.

6th. A bridle, or frœnulum, appears before the lips of the pudendum.

7th. The hymen is likewise present, by which is meant a thin tense membrane, situated at the entrance into the vagina, being sometimes of an oval figure, sometimes circular, and sometimes

sometimes semilunar, and shutting up
the greatest part of the passage. This
hymen hath been esteemed a certain
mark of virginity, when other circumstances concur to give it authority. It
is not, however, by any means absolute, even in the youngest subjects;
for it may be so concealed in the back
of the vagina, as not to be perceptible
at first sight, or it may be destroyed or
obliterated by a variety of causes,
besides a connection with a male. A
fresh rupture of it, however, may be
perceived, and some remains of it will
continue evident for some time.

The marks by which it is most
probable that a female accustomed
herself to venereal habits, and of
consequence is less to be believed
upon a deposition for a rape, are the
following:

Marks of having used venery.

1st. The lips of the pudendum are
flaccid and distended more than in a
maiden.

D   2d.

2d. The clitoris is enlarged, and hath a prepuce which covers the glans arising from constant friction, and is produced to defend it from injuries, in proportion as it is exposed to them.

3d. The nymphæ are likewise enlarged, and are of a lighter and more obscure colour.

4th. The orifice into the urinary passage is more open and exposed. This is owing to the flaccidity of the labiæ.

5th. The hymen is wanting, as may naturally be supposed; but it is not to stand as a test by itself, where the other circumstances do not occur.

6th. Some small excrescences arise in the shape of the berries of the myrtle (called from thence carunculæ myrtiformes) at the entrance into the vagina.

7th. The vagina is enlarged and spacious, and this even where there has been no parturition.

8th.

8th. The wrinkles are less prominent, and in length of time are quite
obliterated.

9th. The orifice of the uterus ap-
proaches nearer than before to the orifice of the vagina. This, however,
must be entirely relative, as the extent
of the vagina must differ in every subject; and besides, it presumes upon
an acquaintance with the person previous to the habit she is engaged in,
which is not easily to be acquired.

CHAP.

CHAP. V.

OF THE MURDER OF INFANTS.

Confined to what ages.

THIS kind of homicide relates to the youngest and most helpless part of the human species, and is confined to them in three states of their existence : just before they are born, at the time of delivery, and immediately, or soon after they are brought into the world. The two last may be included together, and constitute child murder, strictly so called, and the other the murder of a child in its abortive state, or the premature delivery of it so as to procure its death..

State of the mother.

We shall first consider the state of the mother, after she has been delivered of a child, as a leading fact upon which much depends with regard to the destruction either of infants or abortions,

abortions, and then the particular nature of these homicides.

The signs that a woman hath been delivered of a child, are of two kinds, as this circumstance is recent, or has happened for some time back. The signs of the former are, Signs of delivery. Recent.

1st. An extraordinary swelling of the external parts of generation.

2d. A preternatural distension of the vagina.

3d. A flow of the lochia, which is a discharge that differs from the common menstrual flux, in being of a paler colour, and having a sourish disagreeable smell.

4th. The orifice into the uterus is soft and open, as if a late discharge had been made from it; the womb itself too not having properly collapsed and taken its natural shape.

5th. There is a roughness and flaccidity of the abdomen, which is sometimes covered likewise with wrinkles.

6th.

6th. The breasts are swelled to a larger size than common, and are hard and troublesome to the touch, sometimes loaded with excrescences that feel like schirri.

7th. Milk is found in the breasts, which, when curdled, forms the knots above-mentioned, and may be extracted from them by pressure, or by suction.

8th. The nipples become thick and strong, and the disk round them is much widened.

Former.

The signs that a woman hath formerly been delivered of a child, are the following.

1st. All the signs of her having lost her virginity in the last chapter.

2d. The orifice of the womb has not its usual conic figure, and is more open than in a maiden.

3d. The lips of the orifice of the womb are unequal.

4th.

4th. There is a roughness of the abdomen, which is likewise more expanded, and pensile or hanging down.

5th. There are small white and shining lines running on the abdomen.

6th. The frænum of the labiæ pudendi is obliterated.

7th. The breasts are more flaccid and pendulous.

8th. The lines on the breasts are white and splendid.

9th. The colour of the disk is brown.

10th. The nipples are prominent.

11th. There is a prominence of the inner coat of the womb.

12th. There is sometimes an inversion of this body.

The marks of abortion depend on the length of the pregnancy, and must be referred to the judgment of the physician, &c. In general, they are only those of lost virginity.—Vide last chapter.

Marks of abortion.

In

In order to explain those distinctions by which we are to know that an infant, who has been found dead and exposed, was murdered by any inhuman hands or not, we should divide them,

Division of the signs of murder. I. Into those signs by which we know that the child might be born alive, and afterwards be destroyed.

II. Those more evident marks, by which we ascertain that it was brought into the world dead.

III. Those which accurately point out, that force and violence were exercised to deprive it of existence.

IV. Those more particular distinctions which are to be made on a thorough inspection and dissection of the dead body.

Signs that a child was born alive. I. We know that a child has been born alive, when we find that it has exercised any of the vital actions, by which is meant, not those similar actions by which life is supported when

when the fœtus remains in the womb,
but those real actions which are in
force after the child is brought into
the world. These are the circulation
of the blood, and respiration, such as
is enjoyed by animals after their birth.

The following may be esteemed Signs of circulation of blood.
proofs that a child hath enjoyed the
circulation of its blood after it is born;
and thus may be said to be born alive.

1st. The mother, during the whole
state of her pregnancy, must have enjoyed a good state of health, and have
perceived the motions of the infant to
the time of her delivery.

2d. The child, when born, must
be of a proper length and weight.—
Vide chap. ii. p. 15.

3d. The blood vessels of the child
must not be replete with blood.

4th. There must be a settlement of
blood in divers parts of the external
surface of the skin.

5th.

5th. The body of the child must not be rough nor flaccid.

6th. The umbilical cord should be full of juice, and of a white colour.

7th. The placenta, if it be to be found, should be turgid, and its vessels full of blood.

8th. In places that may be pressed in different parts of the body, the blood ought to stagnate, and become coagulated.

9th. A froth should appear upon the mouth of the infant, and stick about its lips.

10th. There should be every appearance of a natural delivery.

It should be remarked here, that these signs should be taken collectively; scarcely any of them will avail when taken separate from each other.

Signs of respiration. The signs that an infant has breathed after it is brought into the world are,

1st.

1st. The act of vociferation after delivery, if positive proof of such a circumstance can be obtained.

2d. The lungs being endued with a colour approaching to a white, being of less specific weight than others, when the child never breathed through them, and being put into water, having a disposition to swim in it. This will be considered more fully.

3d. The lungs are more expanded than in dead subjects; and, previous to delivery, adhere to or rather fill up the cavity of the thorax.

II. The signs by which we can in some measure determine that an infant was brought into the world dead, are to be derived from the following circumstances, and which appear to be of the utmost note. *Signs of an infant being dead.*

1st. When the mother has been for some time afflicted during the time of her pregnancy, with various severe disorders.

D 6   2d.

2d. When she has not perceived for some time the motions of the infant in her womb.

3d. When upon dissection of the head of the infant, the brain appears fluid like water, and has not its usual substance.

4th. When the heart and other blood-vessels are filled with thick and coagulated blood.

5th. When the body of the infant has its flesh collapsed and contracted, its skin soft and flabby, and its whole appearance of a red or scarlet colour.

6th. When compressions on the surface are attended with no *ecchymoses*, or stagnations of blood.

7th. When the blood is of a putrid nature, whilst it continues in the vessels.

8th. When there are evident signs of a putrefaction having taken place, whilst the child was in the womb, such as a separation of the cuticle from the

next

next surface of the skin; the umbilical cord being rotten, wrinkled, of a yellow colour, and as if melting away; a swelling of the abdomen, and a soft tumefaction of the whole body.

9th. When the umbilical cord is not only rotten, but devoid of humours.

10th. When the bones of the skull of the infant are softer and more disjoined than in one born alive.

11th. When other internal parts besides the brain are found corrupted and decayed.

12th. When the *placenta*, or after-birth, at the time of delivery, or soon after, is in a state of corruption.

13th. When there is a defect of the excrement in the large intestines, and of urine in the bladder destined to its use.

14th. When parturition was exceedingly laborious.

15th.

15th. When the lungs are more dense than in a live subject, have a red colour, subside in water when they are thrown into it, and are so collapsed as not to fill up the cavity of the thorax.

16th. When there is an unequal conformation of all the organs destined to their several functions, with respect to length and thickness.

17th. When the little body of the child, if perceived soon after delivery, is not found warm to the feeling.

18th. When the blood flows from the mother in a superabundant quantity, both before and after delivery.

19th. When the mother, during her pregnant state, has been excited to a high degree of anger, or impressed with extraordinary fears.

20th. When she has suffered a great injury during that state, especially in the abdomen.

21st. When at the time of delivery a strong mephitic smell may be
perceived

perceived to issue from the external parts of generation.

22d. When there is a subsidence of the sutures upon the top of the head in the child, without any marks of violent depression.

23d. When the meconium, a kind of fæces, flows from the child at the time of delivery.

A great handle hath been made of the swimming, or subsidence of the lungs. When other circumstances are taken into consideration, it may be a corroborating proof, but can by no means be absolute of itself; for the lungs may swim from putrefaction, where a child is born dead, or from inflation by a blow-pipe, or other means. On the other hand, the lungs may subside in a child that is born alive: for a child may live, or have its circulation perfect, some time before it begins to breathe.

Swimming of lungs examined.

III.

Signs of vi-
olence to
procure
death.

III. We are to consider how to form a judgment, concerning any violence that may have been used to procure the death of a child, and this we derive from the following circumstances.

From
wounds.

1st. When at the time of inspection, marks of certain injuries, such as might have been inflicted upon an adult, as fractures, or wounds, are evident to the senses.

From suf-
focation.

2d. When there are evident marks of suffocation, or strangulation, such as a remarkable compression of the *thorax* or chest; the *aspera arteria,* or wind-pipe being filled with serum or mucus; a redness, or lividity of the countenance; the tongue swelling and prominent; a red, or livid circular line about the neck; the cavities of the mouth and nose full of extraneous matter; a falling in of the flesh about the *scrobiculum cordis,* or pit of the stomach; the lungs livid, filled with blood, and heavier than usual; the

vapours

vapours of sulphur burnt extending to
the lungs; the cavities of the heart,
as the right auricle and ventricle, being filled and expanded with blood;
the jugular veins, and those about the
head, being also distended with blood;
a froth about the mouth; the bladder
empty of urine; the child being found
in places where it is liable to be destroyed by dirt or water, as in ditches
or lakes; and lastly, its being oppressed
soon after delivery by bed-clothes, or
other coverings, which might deprive
it of life.

3d. When there are evident marks Luxation of neck.
of the luxation of the neck, taken not
only from the flaccidity of the head
and neck, but from depressions about
the parts, which are wide and deep.

4th. When there are evident marks Injuries of the skull.
of injuries to the skull, as great depressions and blots near to the sutures,
which arise from extravasations of
blood and serum, and appear either
under

under the skin, or in the hemisphere of the brain, or in its ventricles, or in the base of the skull.

Umbilical cord not tied. 5th. When the umbilical cord does not appear to have been tied, or is entirely torn off from the body. It should be observed, that the neglect of tying the umbilical cord is not always the immediate cause of death to an infant, but only when, from such defect, a mortal hæmorrhage arises, and which may be known,

When the cause of death. 1st. When the whole habit of the body is quite pallid.

2d. When the great blood-vessels, and the cavities of the brain, are empty of blood.

3d. When there is a rupture of the cord in delivery, and the mother has suffered much hæmorrhage both before and after that event.

Circumstances on inspection. IV. It is necessary, perhaps, in many cases where a suspicion of murder is great, but the facts are not so evident,

evident, to exercise the judgment as
well as the observation of the person
employed to give a deposition. And
here are some rules necessary to be observed to execute his intention in a
masterly, judicious, and accurate manner. In the first place, he should consider, whether the body be in a state of
putrefaction, or not, and whether that Putrefaction.
putrefaction is in such degree as to
preclude all observation. If that be
not the case, perhaps an examination
may be made upon the bones of the
head, or other parts, so far as to
ascertain,

1st. Whether the fœtus be of mature growth; and this may be known
from the size as well as the conformation of them.

2d. Whether such violences have
been used as to injure these parts, as
by fractures, &c.

If a degree of putrefaction has not
taken place, so far as to preclude our
observation,

observation, the rules may be divided into those that relate to the inspection, and those that relate to the dissection of the body.

When a proper inspection is made, we should examine,

Clothes. 1st. Whether the clothes in which the child is wrapped up be tinged with blood, or whether there be any blood upon the external surface of the skin.

Sex and growth. 2d. Of what sex the child is, and whether it be come to mature growth.

Superficies of the body. 3d. The whole superficies of the body is to be examined from head to foot, to see whether there are any *ecchymoses*, or stagnations of blood; livid spots, or spots of various colours; whether the skin itself be grown livid, with or without any signs of violence, or other injuries, such as punctures in the head or neck, luxations, and subsidence of the sutures, with or without any violent depression.

4th.

4th. The heat of the face, in particular, and of the whole body, are to be attended to. And here we must guard against deception, for a dead fœtus may partake in some measure of the heat of the mother; so that if a dead fœtus were to be examined immediately after delivery, and a child born alive, some little time after death, they might both enjoy the same degree of heat. Other circumstances then here must be taken into the account. *Heat of the child,*

5th. The cavities of the mouth and nose are to be examined, to see whether any foreign matter is deposited in them. This cannot be, unless the child had enjoyed life so far as to open these passages. We should observe likewise, whether it has grasped any thing in its hands, as this is a certain proof of life. *Cavities.*

6th. We should examine the umbilical cord, whether it adhere to the *Umbilical cord.*

placenta,

placenta, if it be tied, or is broken, or cut off, and what is its colour, and what its length.

Placenta, 7th. The *placenta*, or after-birth, likewise should be examined, to see whether it adhere to the umbilical cord; whether it be dry or moist, and how far it may have become schirrous.

Appearances on dissection. We are next to consider, what is to be done upon a dissection of the body, and this ought never to be omitted: and here the following rules should be observed.

Principal cavities to be opened. 1st. All the three principal cavities of the body, the head, the *thorax* or chest, and the *abdomen* or belly, should be opened, to discover any injuries that may have happened to the substances contained in them, and the great vessels which run through them.

Lungs examined. 2d. The lungs should be properly examined, and every enquiry made into their colour, connection, density,

density, substance, and specific gravity;
and whether they may not be indurated
in some places, and how far they exhi‑
bit signs of putrefaction.

3d. The *aspera arteria*, or wind‑ Wind‑
pipe, should be cut through, to disco‑ pipe.
ver how far it is filled with mucus or
serum. The great vessels, and the ca‑
vities of the heart likewise, should be
opened, not only to observe how far
they are full or empty of blood, but
that the colour and consistence of that
fluid may be ascertained. Having
made these observations, the lungs,
with the heart are to be cut out of the
body. After this the heart is to be se‑
parated from them, and the vessels
tied ! they are then to be thrown into a
large bason of moderately warm water,
and it is to be observed how far they
sink or swim in it. After this, each
tube of the lungs is to be examined se‑
parately, and the same observations to
be made upon it.

4th.

4th. All the other viscera, but particularly those of the abdomen, are to be examined, but the great intestines especially, to see whether they are full of meconium, and the bladder if it be exhausted of urine.

We cannot help lamenting here, that although so much is required, so little is generally done in these cases; and that an innocent life is often sacrificed to hurry, to negligence, or ignorance; whilst a wretch, who is devoid of shame, escapes from punishment, for want of judgment, accuracy and attention. And it is to be hoped, that this little treatise will meet the attention of judges and lawyers in this particular circumstance, which so often comes before them, to the shame and scandal of humanity; and that they will be enabled to correct the errors of coroners, or ignorant surgeons, who may have been misled in the depositions they give in. It is a misfortune, tine, that men of eminence in the physical line fly from bars of judicature, as places of trouble and examination. It may be necessary, therefore, to give the court such checks upon ignorance, as will serve to discover the truth.

The next thing to be considered Abortion before we finish this chapter, is with respect to abortions, or the destruction of those unborn embryos which were never brought into the world: and indeed as such beings might live, and become of use to mankind, and as they may be supposed from the time indeed of conception, to be living animated beings, there is no doubt but the destruction of them ought to be considered as a capital crime. It is neces- No medi- sary then, that we enquire whether any cine can procure it, medicines can be given, or other means used, absolutely to procure this effect; and indeed it is evident, I believe, from experience, that such

E   things

things cannot act as efficient causes,
without the aid of those predisposing
causes, or natural habits of the body,
which are necessary to concur with
them. As attempts of this kind,
however, should not be passed off with
impunity, and as the life of the mother, as well [as the child, is endan-
gered by such exhibitions, if advised
by any other, they should be considered
as highly culpable, and for this reason
should be made known.

Methods generally used.

The common methods made use of
are the stronger vomits and purges,
venæsection to a great degree, all that
class of medicines called emmenagogues, and those which have a ten-
dency to promote salivation. External methods are, irritations of the
mouth of the womb, strong passions of
the mind, painful disorders, fevers, &c.
The predisposing causes must be,
great fulness of the blood, irritability
of the womb, a defect in the nutriment

ment of the fœtus, a womb that will not suffer itself to be distended beyond a certain degree, and a morbid disposition of the placenta.

It is to be lamented here too, that whilst this crime, which is practised generally by the most abandoned, escapes unpunished, a poor deluded creature, in the case of infant murder, whose shame highly extenuates her guilt, should suffer death, where nature had acted so forcibly as almost to overcome her fatal resolutions, and had taken away all power to put in practice the subtle contrivances of art.

CHAP.

CHAP. VI.

ON HOMICIDE.

Nature of man. THAT wonderful machine of which human nature is composed, which is directed and ordered by a contrivance unknown to the wisest of men, and which gives birth to all our pleasures and enjoyments, contains nothing in itself to perpetuate its own existence. A very little derangement of its functions, or of its acting principles, will deprive it of life, and destroy all its **How deprived of life.** powers of action. The most common methods by which men lose their **By disease.** lives, are by diseases which are generally, though impiously, attributed to the hand of God: for what we incur by our own vices and imprudence, what by the passions and evil dispositions of others preying upon our spirits, and what by bad customs and habits,

bits, we must attribute more of death to any other cause, than what is assigned. Where death is occasioned in any other manner than by disease, it is called natural, where it arises from some accident, which shall immediately cause a dissolution of our powers ; or homicide where it is effected by the violent hand of another. In such a case, the law justly retaliates upon the offender, where it is committed from anger and malice, and is not, as in the case of war, protected by the sovereign influence of princes.

Where it comes under the cognizance of a court of judicature, the greatest circumspection and attention are required, and the laws of all countries have appointed proper officers previous to any trial; and as soon as possible after the murder, to enquire into the causes and nature of it, how it was committed, and what appearances present themselves upon inspection.

Natural cause.

Homicide.

Officers to enquire.

E 3   In

Directions how to examine.

In the exmination which is made, (before a decision be pronounced), the following directions are necessary to be observed.

When to be made, and where.

I. The examination of the dead body should be as soon as possible after death, in the day time, at a proper place, where a dissection, if necessary, (and it is almost always necessary) may be performed, and not according to vulgar custom, where it is found, let it be ever so improper, and likewise by proper instruments, such as are generally used by surgeons in their dissections, and not by coarse and rude knives and scissars, which may mangle and tear the body, but cannot ascertain the cause of its death.

Accurate inspection of sound body.

II. Before a dissection be proposed, a very accurate inspection should be made upon the sound body, in order to discover how far the death was occasioned by suffocation from mineral vapours, the fermentation of new liquor,

quor, the burning of charcoal, or the electric shock of lightning. In such cases, except the last, and then they do not seem to be the cause of the death, no marks are to be found.

III. Upon a further inspection, it is to be examined, 1st. into any deviations from the natural state of the external superficies of the body, as whether there are any spots which are derived from the blood's escaping into vessels not fitted to convey it; ecchymoses, which are stagnations arising under the skin, or pericranium of the head; or any other spots in the external surface; and of these we are to examine the situation, magnitude, figure and number. We must examine likewise, under this head, the nature of any tumours which may appear, and whether they are owing to violence, or any other cause: their size and figure should also be described. And, lastly, we should enquire into the state of

Spots on the body.

Tumours.

E 4   putrefaction

Putrefac-
tion.

putrefaction of the body, which is known by the following particulars. 1st. Bladders filled with a yellow or brownish liquor. 2d. The external cuticle separated from the true skin. 3d. A lividity and blackness of the skin. 4th. A fœtor, or disagreeable smell of the whole body. 5th. A considerable swelling of the carcase. 6th. A particular lividity and blackness in the scrotum of male subjects. 7th. A blackness of the nails.

wounds,
&c.

2d. Into any wounds which are conspicuous, and remark whether they be over the whole body, or confined to a particular part; and here no probe or other instrument should be inserted which may enlarge them, and alter their nature.

Blood or
other hu-
mour flow-
ing from
carcase.

3d. Whether from the carcase in general, or from any wound or aperture, as the mouth, anus, &c. there be a flowing of blood, urine, or meconium.

4th.

4th. Into the habit of the body, whether it be fat or lean, or swelled from any cause. Habit of body.

IV. The directions to be attended under a dissection are the following. Dissection.

1st. The integuments of the body, and especially of those places which require examination, where any wounds present, are to be dissected away, and the muscles are to be cut through, in order to open a way to the parts where injury is supposed to be done. Integuments.

2d. All the chief cavities of the body, as the head, the chest, and the belly, are to be opened. Cavities.

2d. That cavity is to be penetrated first where the injury is supposed to reside. Where injury received.

4th. The parts circumjacent to a wound are not to be dissected before the progress of the injury is traced to its utmost extent. Parts circumjacent.

5th. Any bowel contained in the cavity, is to be examined according to Bowels.

its situation, connections, constitution, and any wounds which it may have received, in their length, breadth, and depth.

Fore'gn bo-
dies.

6th. We should enquire if the bowel opened contain any foreign bodies, either fluid or solid: if the former, their nature and quantity is to be determined; if the latter, their quality, number, quantity, figure, and situation.

Blood ves-
sels.

7th. All the great blood vessels passing through a cavity, are to be examined whether they be entire or no, and whether they contain blood or not.

Nerves,
&c.

8th. The great nerve likewise, as the *medulla spinalis*, or spinal marrow, &c. should undergo an examination, and the thoracic duct and receptacle of the chyle, vessels which carry the nutriment from the stomach, and from the external surface into the mass of blood.

9th.

9th. Before the head be opened, it Head opened. should be discovered whether there are any wounds in the skull by fracture, fissure, intropression, &c. and of such the situation, size, depth, number, and figure should be marked.

10th. When the head is opened, Skull. the skull should be carefully taken off with a saw.

11th. When the brain is exa- Brain. mined, regard must be had to its substance, to its vessels, whether they be full or empty of blood; to the sinusses of the dura mater, those large receptacles of blood which lie under the skull; to the ventricles or cavities, to see whether any fluid be contained in them, and of what nature, and in what quantity; to the base of the skull, to discover if any foreign body lies upon it; and lastly, to the thickness of the bones, whether it be ordinary or extraordinary.

E 6 12th.

Chest. .12th. When the chest is opened, the sternum is to be separated from the ribs with great care, lest the arteries or veins lying near it, or in the cavity, be injured.

Ribs. 13th. If a wound should be made in the chest, and which penetrates either side, then we should not only determine the ribs between which the wound is made, but from whence we reckon.

Heart. . 14th. When the heart is examined we should take notice, whether polypous concretions occur in its cavities, or in the greater vessels.

Rupture of bowels. 15th. When a rupture of any of the bowels is discovered upon dissection, we should carefully examine whether it be recent, or whether it be gangrenous, or have the signs of putrefaction.

Contents of bowels of abdomen. 16th. When the bowels of the lower belly, which are large cavities, are submitted to examination, we should

should enquire with the utmost care into their contents, and this not only by simple inspection, but by the fire and chemical mixtures.

There are besides these, some other circumstances to be attended to, as the constitution of the dead person, the instrument by which his death was occasioned, the symptoms under which he laboured, the means used to restore him, the time when assistance was called to him, his situation when wounded, his diet before and after, and lastly, whether he was affected with drunkenness.

The different kinds of murder, or the different means by which it is committed, may be reduced to poisons, wounds, bruises, drowning, and strangulation. The two first seem to be the most common; the third is often rather a remote than a proximate cause, and the two others are chiefly discovered by the facts, rather than

by

by any peculiar marks they leave on the body. But first of poisons.

Of poisons defined.

A poison may be defined any substance, which, applied to the human body internally, is injurious to its preservation, or procures its dissolution by its own proper qualities. The

Ways by which they act,

ways by which poisons get into the body, are by the mouth, nose, lungs, and sometimes the external surface of the skin, and these modes of action may be explained in the following manner.

Mode of action.

Health supposes a natural state or constitution of the fluids and solids of the animal body. All poisons then, must act in destroying this natural constitution of parts, and changing it into a preternatural one. There are various ways by which this is done; the principal are the following.

By acrids.

1st. By acrid things, which constringe and erode the solids, or sometimes

times coagulate, sometimes resolve the fluids.

2d. When they possess a power of stupefying or destroying the powers of sensation and motion in the nerves, which are the great agents of the animal machine. *Stupefyers.*

3d. When they possess a sharp and acute figure, which tears and lancinates the tender parts of the stomach and bowels. *Figure sharp.*

4th. When they induce a powerful suffocation. *Suffocation.*

5th. When they act not only from acrimony, but from a power of thickening the blood at the same time. *Tenacity.*

6th. When they have the power of thickening and of drying also the humours. *Drying.*

7th. When they act by some unknown power, which is not yet discovered. *Unknown power.*

It would be useless, nay perhaps injurious to society, to enumerate all the

the poisons which belong to the different heads. It is dangerous to entrust
such materials in the hands of mankind in general : we hope, therefore,
we shall be excused if we mention only
the principal ones, according to the
foregoing arrangement. They are all
taken from the animal, vegetable, and
mineral kingdoms.

Acrids
what.

The 1st class or acrids, include
acids, and alcalies ; among the last of
which may be included the effects of
the putrefactive process, as being exposed to its influence.

Those poisons of an acrid nature
which have a mixed quality, are the
metallic salts, or some of the semi-me-
tals themselves, as arsenic, &c. and
some vegetables which are of a highly
drastic nature, and which, used in
small quantities, may produce useful
evacuations in cases of disease.

Stupefy-
ers.

2d. The poisons which have a stupefying quality are of the vegetable
kind, as the Cicuta, lauro cerasus, &c.

3d.

3d. Those which act mechanically by the sharp points and edges with which they are endued, are the powder of glass, diamonds, &c. Mechanic powers.

4th. Those which have a suffocating power, are the vapours of new and fermenting liquors, the smoke of charcoal and of sulphur, the air of close and damp places, &c. Suffocations.

5th. Those which have a viscidity joined with acrimony, are generally vegetables, such as Cicuta major, solanum, &c. Viscid.

6th. Those which are of a thickening quality, and a drying one at the same time, are quick-lime, Cerusse; and among the vegetables, several of the class of fungi, &c. Dryers.

7th. Those which have a secret quality, not easily discovered, are the various tribes of animals which live around us, such as spiders, toads, vipers, &c. Unknown qualities.

The

How poisons affect the body.

The effects which poisons produce upon the body vary, according to the nature of their qualities, the place which they affect, and the subjects to whom they are applied, according to age, temperament, habit of body, &c.

Aconite. Thus the aconite affects the lips, mouth, forehead, tongue and stomach, by making them to swell, and causes anxieties, vertigoes, faintings, and convulsions.

Cicuta. The cicuta occasions enormous vomitings, hiccups, heat of the stomach, swelling of the belly, delirium, and convulsions.

Acids The acid spirits, wherever they touch, cause erosions, most grievous

Arsenic, &c. pains, vomiting, and hiccup. Arsenic and cobalt excite inflammations of the stomach, &c. the most acute pains, heat in the mouth and jaws, nausea or sickness, vomiting, spasmodic contractions of the chest, swelling of the belly,

belly, coldness of the extremities, cold sweats, convulsions, &c.

When a medical practitioner therefore, is called to a person who is suspected to be poisoned, if he be alive, he may judge from the following observations. How to judge in a living subject.

1st. From comparing the symptoms which present themselves with those which generally attend the taking of poisons mentioned above. From symptoms above.

2d. From the sudden appearance of some symptoms, such as spasms and violent pains, great thirst, sickness, vomiting, fainting, cholic, the throwing up some foreign matter from the general contents of the stomach, and universal convulsion of all the muscles. From suddenness of some symptoms.

3d. From the health of the patient foregoing this attack, and his not having any connection with a person labouring under any contagious or epidemic disease. Previous health.

4th.

No errors
in diet.
4th. From the patient having committed no errors in diet, &c.

From
odour and
taste.
5th. From an ungrateful odour and taste of what has been taken. There are few poisons but what are attended with a very disagreeable smell and taste; hence a suspicion soon arises from this source, which if immediately taken notice of, the patient may soon receive the proper relief.

How to
judge in a
dead person.
But if the person be dead, a very minute examination must be made, and the following particulars attended to.

From external habit.
1st. The external habit of the body is to be inspected with the greatest accuracy and attention, to discover whether there be any livid spots upon the surface of the skin; whether there are any premature signs of putrefaction, and whether there be any swelling of the belly, or of the face; for experience evinces that these changes

are

are soon induced by poisonous substances.

2d. The passages by which the poi- The passages.
son has been conveyed into the body,
are to be examined: these are the
mouth, the throat or gullet, the sto-
mach, and the intestines; but chiefly Principally the stomach.
the stomach, as the same effects will
be produced in it as in the other
parts. We must examine then first
into its constitution, and then into its
contents.

When we examine the constitution In its constitution.
or form of the stomach, we must
consider,

1st. Whether it be inflated or cor-
rugated in an extraordinary manner.

2d. Whether it be inflamed, or in a
state of gangrene or mortification.

3d. Whether it exhibits upon its
external surface supernatural spots,
either of a red colour, or black or livid.

4th. Whether it be perforated into
holes, either one or many.

5th.

5th. Whether its veins be tinged with blood more than usual.

5th. Whether it be eroded, and its inner coat be stripped off and bloody, and swim amongst the other contents.

7th. Whether there be any eschar in its substance, of a black or yellowish colour.

All these marks afford very strong suspicions of poisons, especially of those which are acute and acrid.

Contents of the stomach.

The next observations are to be made upon the contents of the stomach, previous to which two circumstances must be attended to.

1st. All the contents of the stomach are to be thrown into a vessel prepared for that purpose.

2d. The surface of the stomach is to be inspected more carefully, to discover, if possible, whether particles of the poison may not stick to it, which are to be collected.

The

The contents of the stomach are to be considered as more or less fluid; if they are not entirely so, but consist of many solid substances, then a por- tion of them is to be dried and put into an iron vessel lined with tin, and being previously weighed, the follow- ing experiments are to be made upon it. *Solid.*

1st. It is to be thrown upon burn- ing coals; which, if it produces a va- pour of a blue colour, and an odour like that of garlic is perceived, it may be nearly ascertained that an arsenical matter was mixed with it. But in or- der to clear up this point to greater satisfaction. *To be tried by burn- ing.*

2d. Another portion of the dried mass is to be given to other animals, such as fowls, dogs, &c. which, if it causes their death, it is a proof that poison made a part of its contents. *By other animals.*

3d. Another portion of this dried mass is to be mixed with a quantity of *Mixed with suet and sal. tart. and melt- ed.*

of suet and salt of tartar, which being put into a crucible, and melted over the fire, if a reguline metallic substance is produced at the bottom, it is clear that an arsenic is contained in it.

Melted with other metals.

4th. It may be enquired, whether this metallic substance being melted again with metals of a red colour, turn them to a white, for this is likewise proof of arsenic.

Remainder weighed.

The remainder of the dried contents, if poison be found upon experiment, must be nicely and accurately weighed. This is to discover, whether the proportionate quantity would be sufficient to produce the effect. But in general, where arsenic has been administered, so small a quantity is sufficient to produce the most dreadful influence, that it will be nearly satisfactory, if any of it be found upon a chemical examination.

When

When the fluid parts of the stomach are examined, the following experiments are to be made. Fluid parts examined.

1st. An alcaline liquor, as oil of tartar per delinquium, for instance, is to be thrown in, and if it take a brownish colour, it is a proof that mercury, in the shape of corrosive sub-limate, or precipitate, has been mixed with it, if it ferments, that an acid has been exhibited. This, however, is no certain sign, as an acid may subsist very innocently in the stomach. By alcalines.

2d. An acid may be applied, and here, if an effervescence be produced, it is a proof of an alcaline substance, and then, as in the last case, it must be by the quantity and acrimony of the substances that we determine concerning their poisonous nature, as in themselves, and when well diluted, they arc innocent and sometimes salutary. By acids.

F   3d.

By colour.
3d. The colour is likewise to be attended to, as it may determine the exact nature of the poison which is given.

By chemical analysis.
4th. Some portion of the poison found may be sent to a chemical elaboratory, to examine more particularly its nature.

These observations, it should be remarked, however, relate more particularly to poisons which produce their effect more immediately, than to those which lie a long time first, in the stomach. But we may, from the injuries done to the stomach itself, determine likewise in some measure concerning even those more slowly acting poisons. The remains of inflammation, gangrene, perforations, &c. will continue for a long time, and if the patient should die of poison at ever so great a distance, whilst the cause subsists some effect will evidently be perceived,

ceived, or some change from a natural state.

2d. Of wounds. Under wounds may be comprehended every disorder which arises from some external violence offered to the human body. To this head, therefore, may belong contusions, luxations, fractures, and wounds, more properly so called, being a division of the muscular parts of the body. The first division of wounds is into mortal, and the contrary. Every wound is of such a nature, that death is absolutely the consequence of it or not. In the latter case it may be called mortal by accident. This also we may divide into two kinds or orders. That wound which is so inflicted that it may be relieved by the means cognizable by art, is of the first order. That where it happens that the death which is incurred, is owing not to the wound, but to other causes, then the

F 2   wound

Wounds defined.

Division.

Mortal what.

Mortal by accident.

wound is said to be of the second order of such as are called mortal by accident.

From what hath been advanced, the following positions may be deduced.

Positions. 1st. Every wound, absolutely mortal, will admit of no relief, but will certainly destroy, either by a sudden or lingering death.

2d. Death is always the inseparable effect of a wound absolutely mortal.

3d. A wound absolutely mortal is always the *sole* cause of death to the injured person.

4th. The consequences here avail nothing: the wounded person, after the wound is inflicted, is to all intents and purposes a dead man; the injury then is absolutely mortal.

5th. Wounds are by accident mortal, when the cause of death arises
partly

partly from the wound, and partly from other concurring causes.

These distinctions are necessary, though not always attended to ; for it may so happen, where men judge alone from consequences, that a person may be punished for a death occasioned by a wound which was not absolutely mortal. It is highly important that in a deposition for murder, such distinctions should be made of these kinds of wounds, as to place them in their proper light. In order to do this more effectually, it is necessary to make the following divisions. 1st. To consider those kinds of wounds which are absolutely mortal, or mortal by accident. 2d, In what parts of the body such wounds are most likely to be inflicted. 3d. Some circumstances which may occur to distinguish such wounds more accurately.

I. It appears then, that because a mortal wound cannot be cured by

Reasons for such distinctions.

Division of rules.

What kind of wounds mortal.

F 3   any

any art, that every wound which entirely takes off the influx of the blood into the heart, from the vein, and its egress from the heart into the arteries, or which entirely destroys the powers of circulation, and the action of the heart, must be absolutely mortal. From the elements of physiology it appears, that the following circumstances are necessary to promote the action of the heart.

Actions of the heart promoted by.

1st. The soundness of the sides of the cavities of the heart, so as to be able not only to contain the blood, but to push it forward into the system. The strength required here is amazingly great.

Soundness of walls.

2d. A free action of the brain and nerves going to the heart, called the cardiac nerves.

Action of the brain.

3d. The motion of the blood through the coronary arteries which surround the heart.

Coronary arteries.

4th.

4th. A free motion of the blood Lungs. through the lungs.

5th. A proper return of blood Proper return. through the veins.

6th. A renewal by the aliment of Aliment. nutriment to restore the expence which is incurred by the several secretions, &c. It appears then that all wounds Mortal in are absolutely mortal. that order.

1st. Which injure the cavities of the heart, so that they cannot contain the blood.

2d. Which take away the free action of the brain and nerves going to the heart, so that neither sense nor motion can be promoted in that organ so essential to life.

3d. Which destroy respiration, for then the blood cannot be carried through the lungs.

4th. Which stop the motion of the blood through the coronary arteries.

5th. Which prevent its return through the veins.

F 4   6th.

· 6th. Which prevent the use of nutriment, and consequently the accession of chyle.

It appears then, that the subject of wounds absolutely mortal are those parts whose soundness cannot be taken away, and life continue; and that many of those wounds which happen in internal parts, to which the medical aid cannot reach, are to be considered as absolutely mortal.

Wounds mortal by accident. When a wound is mortal by accident, death is either to be attributed to it in part as a concurring circumstance, or not at all: as in such cases as the following.

When left to themselves. 1st. Where death is occasioned by wounds being left to themselves, as for instance, wounds of the head which may be cured by the use of the trepan; those of the greater blood vessels, where access may be acquired; those of the viscera, where the hand may be applied, and medicines may be administered;

nistered; those which induce death by evacuations into cavities, which might be prevented, or from which they may easily be discharged.

2d. Where other causes may be the occasion of death, as the particular constitution, or habit of the wounded person, as well as his neglect and want of prudence, the fault of the medical practitioner, the blunders and carelessness of by-standers, or some previous disorders which may have prevailed.

Where there are other causes.

II. We are now to consider the second general division, or those wounds of the different parts of the body which are to be accounted mortal absolutely or not; and here we shall treat of them in the following order: 1st. Wounds of the head and neck. 2d. Wounds of the chest. 3d. Wounds of the abdomen or belly. 4th. Wounds of the extremities.

Parts where wounds are mortal or not.

I.

I. Of wounds of the head.——
These are external or internal, which may be again distinguished according to any injury done to the brain, &c. or not.

Of the head.

1st. External wounds of the head, whether they are wounds of the integuments, or of the pericranium, or of the bones composing the skull, or of the face, are not absolutely mortal.

External

2d. Internal wounds of the head, unaccompanied with injuries of the brain, &c. are not to be accounted absolutely mortal.

Internal.

3d. Those wounds of the inner part of the head, where the brain, &c. likewise is injured, are to be accounted absolutely mortal, or not, according to the following distinctions.

Where brain, &c. affected.

1st. Wounds of the dura mater, where there is no sinus or branch of the greater artery running across it that is injured, are not absolutely mortal.

2d.

2d. Wounds of the dura mater in
its sinus, and the greater artery, are to
be accounted absolutely mortal.

3d. All wounds of the contents of
the skull, which are attended with
great extravasations of humours which
cannot be evacuated: as in the ventricles of the brain, and the base of
the skull, are to be accounted absolutely mortal; such are, what are made
at the bottom of the skull, in the bones
of the temples, the ethmoid bones, and
the inferior orbits of the eyes.

4th. Slight wounds of the brain
itself, or of the superficial part of the
cerebellum, are not absolutely mortal.

5th. All wounds of the cerebellum,
which are deep, and of the medulla
oblongata, are accounted absolutely
mortal.

6th. All injuries of the origin of the
spinal marrow, and all deep wounds
through its whole length, may be pronounced absolutely mortal.

With

With regard to wounds of the neck, we may make the following observations.

Wounds of the neck.

1st. Wounds of the internal jugular veins are absolutely mortal; those of the external, only so by accident.

Internal jugular veins.

2d. Wounds of the carotid and vertebral arteries, may be pronounced absolutely mortal.

Carotid arteries.

3d. Wounds of the internal maxillary artery, and the sublingual artery, belong to those esteemed absolutely mortal, if they cannot be healed.

Internal maxillary.

4th. Wounds of the branches of the carotid artery, which can be tied or compressed so as to stop the blood, may be accounted mortal by accident.

Branches of carotid.

5th. Wounds of the intercostal nerves, and of the parvagum, and of the phrenic nerves, which run through the neck, induce absolute death.

Intercostal nerves, &c.

6th.

6th. Wounds of that plexus of nerves which reaches from the spinal marrow to the arm, are the causes of death.

From spinal marrow to arm

7th. All luxations of the first and second vertebræ bring absolute death.

Luxations.

8th. Small wounds of the œsophagus, or gullet, are only mortal by accident; but if the gullet be cut through, they are amongst those which are accounted absolutely mortal.

Œsophagus.

9th. In the same manner slight wounds of the *aspera arteria*, or windpipe, belong to those which are mortal by accident; but if it be cut through, they are always mortal.

Windpipe.

10th. All violent strokes upon the *larynx*, or cartilaginous muscles, on the top of the wind-pipe, so as to destroy their tone and power of action, will speedily induce the death of the sufferer.

Larynx.

II.

II. **Wounds** of the chest are of two kinds, as they are made in the cavity, or in the parts surrounding it. Of the former,

Wounds of chest.

1st. All wounds of the heart, which penetrate into its cavities, *i. e.* into its ventricles, or auricles, are absolutely mortal. The same may be said,

Heart.

2d. Of all wounds of the coronary arteries, which surround the heart, and all the great arteries and veins which carry blood from the heart, and bring it back again.

Coronary arteries.

3d. Wounds of the intercostal arteries, or small vessels which pass between the ribs, are only mortal by accident.

Intercostal arteries.

4th. Wounds of that part of the gullet which lies in the chest, are absolutely mortal. The same may be said,

Gullet.

5th. Of wounds of the wind-pipe in the same situation.

Wind-pipe.

6th.

6th. All wounds of the pericardium, *Pericardium.* or bag containing the heart, are not absolutely mortal.

7th. Wounds of the lungs, which *Lungs.* pierce the great blood-vessels, are absolutely mortal; but those which penetrate the smaller vessels, are only accidentally so.

8th. Wounds of the air vessels of *Bronchia.* any magnitude, are absolutely mortal.

9th. Superficial wounds of the muscular part of the diaphragm, or midriff, *Diaphragm.* are mortal only by accident; but those which pierce the tendinous are absolutely so.

10th. Injuries to the thoracic duct, *Thoracic duct.* which convey the chyle, are mortal absolutely, as are,

11th. Those of the cardiac nerves, *Cardiac nerves.* &c.

II. Wounds made upon the parts surrounding the chest, are to be judged *Surrounding the chest.* by the following decisions:

1st.

1st. All external wounds of the chest are not absolutely mortal.

2d. A simple luxation or fracture of the ribs, is not absolutely mortal.

3d. Considerable bruises, and injuries of the walls of the chest, with dilacerations of the intercostal arteries, are absolutely mortal.

4th. A wound of the chest, where one side only is penetrated in a certain place, is mortal by accident.

5th. Every wound which is of any size, that pierces both sides of the cavity of the chest, is absolutely mortal.

As the chest is the seat of the great fountain of blood, it is no wonder that any injuries committed there should be mortal, and even in those cases where the exceptions are made, the hæmorrhage of itself may cause death.

Wounds of the abdomen. III. Wounds of the abdomen, or lower belly, are judged by the following rules.

1st.

1st. Every wound of the abdomen which does not penetrate into its cavity, whether it be a wound of the integuments, or of the muscles, or of the *linea alba*, as it is called, or of the navel, or of the abdominal ring, are not absolutely mortal, nor are they such when they do penetrate the cavity, when none of the contents are injured.

2d. Wounds of the *omentum*, or caul, where its blood-vessels are hurt, so that the haemorrhage cannot be restrained by any art, are absolutely mortal, otherwise they are mortal only by accident. Omentum,

3d. Wounds of the stomach are absolutely mortal, when many of the nerves are at the same time injured, when some of the principal blood-vessels are cut through, or they are made in such a place, that the food cannot arrive at the hollow part of it, but is thrown into the cavity of the abdomen. Stomach.

men. The same may be observed where the bottom or curvature of it is wounded, or it is pushed to one side.

Small intestines. 4th. A wound in the small intestines, so as to separate them from the stomach, is absolutely mortal.

Great intestines. 5th. Wounds of the great, as well as small intestines, at some distance from the stomach, which do not divide the tube, are not absolutely mortal.

Liver if great. 6th. Wounds of the liver, which are deep and broad, and are supposed to be connected with injuries done to the large vessels passing through it, are absolutely mortal; in like manner are any wounds of the duct of the liver, of the cystic duct, of the gall-bladder, of the *ductus choledochus*, of the vena portarum, or of the artery of the liver.

Small wounds of liver. 7th. Slight wounds of the liver, which do not occasion an extravasation of the humours, are mortal only by accident.

8th.

8th. A rupture of the liver is always absolutely mortal. Rupture of liver.

9th. Deep and broad wounds of the spleen are absolutely mortal, as well as a rupture of the spleen, but slight wounds are only mortal by accident. Spleen.

10th. All wounds of the receptacle of the chyle are absolutely mortal; the same may be pronounced of Receptacle of chyle.

11th. All the great vessels, arteries, and veins, and the nerves which run through the abdomen. Great vessels.

12th. Wounds of the *pancreas*, or milt, as the trunks of many large vessels pass through it, are absolutely mortal. The same may be said, Pancreas.

13th. Of wounds of the mesentery, or external covering of the bowels, for the same reasons, upon account of the vessels. Mesentery.

14th. Wounds of the kidney which reach to the bosom of it, and cut off the ureters, are absolutely mortal; slighter ones are only so by accident. Kidneys

15th.

Bladder.   15th. Wounds of the urinary bladder, where the blood cannot be stopped, are absolutely mortal, and no excuse can be made here from wounds being inflicted by surgical operations. Such being immediately under the eye of the operator, can be easily restrained, so as to have no ill effect.

Genitals in men.   16th. Wounds of the external parts of generation in men, in which may be included contusions of the testicles, are not absolutely mortal.

Womb.   17th. Wounds of the womb are absolutely mortal.

Extremities.   IV.. Wounds of the extremities in general are not absolutely mortal, but sometimes they are, as when they are made upon the trunks of the largest vessels, in which case such an hæmorrhage may arise, as no art can restrain, or from the vital powers being weakened, a most powerful and fatal gangrene or mortification may be occasioned,

sioned, and so as to elude the force of medicines.

III. We come now to the last division of rules, concerning wounds, to examine some circumstances by which the mortality of their nature may be more exactly ascertained. These relate,

1st. To the wounded person himself, in whom we should attend to his age, his constitution of body, his exemption from former injuries, or his subjection to disease, the sex, and if a woman, whether she be pregnant or not; the state of his mind, and how far his imagination might increase the efficacy of the wound; and lastly, whether he was at the time inebriated with liquor. All these circumstances aggravate the mortality of wounds.

2d. To the symptoms which occur, either immediately upon a person's being wounded, or which appear some time after; the symptoms besides these may be of three kinds.

1st.

1st. Those which acknowledge the wound to be their sole cause.

2d. Which depend upon the wound partly as their cause.

3d. Which do not acknowledge the wound to be their cause at all. Now in reviewing the symptoms, it will appear that the first alone are objects of attention.

Instrument.

3d. To the instrument with which the injury was effected, in which its figure, its size, its power of acting, are to be taken into consideration.

Time.

4th. To the time when death may occur after the wound is given.

Cure.

5th. To the methods made use of to effect a cure.

Exposure.

6th. To many occurrences which may arise from the circumstances of time; and any other accidents which might render a wound more dangerous, such as cold air, or a desert place, where no one might be ready to assist.

CHAP.

CHAP. VII.

OF IDIOTISM AND INSANITY.

WHEN the ideas of the mind are distracted, and thought and reason are confused and destroyed; it is common for the civil power, not only to take cognizance of the unhappy persons subject to such misfortunes, but to deprive them of their estates for a time; and put them under proper confinement. As the consequences are so dreadful, it is necessary then that the decision be established upon the firmest and most satisfactory proof.

Idiotism and insanity, though punished in the same manner, seem to vary from each other. It may be necessary then to specify the proper distinctions of each.

Objects of civil power

How distinguished.

1.

I. Idiotism is 1st, either born with the subject of it, or appears as soon as the reasoning faculties should begin to expand.

Idiotism natural.

2d. It is established upon great defects of the memory, and much greater of the judgment, though this is not much attended to.

Depends on defects in memory and judgment.

3d. Idiots are in general prone to mischief, or to actions over which reason seems to have very little command.

Prone to mischief.

4th. They have not a proper command over the evacuation of fæces and urine, and drivel at the mouth.

Insensible to evacuations.

5th. They have generally strong and hearty constitutions.

Health.

6th. They have a peculiar aspect, which describes a vacancy of thought and inattention to any engagement.

Aspect peculiar.

7th. They have little use of speech, and articulate very incoherently.

Inarticulation.

II. Insane persons are either furious or melancholie, both of which acknowledge a great imbecility of the mental

Insanity cause of.

mental faculties, and which are derived from hereditary constitutions, attention of mind, violent passions, the terrors of a false religion, immoderate use of venery, poisons of the narcotic kind, some preceding disorders, the suppression of evacuations, indigestible aliments, a sedentary life, &c. But they differ in the following particulars.

1st. The furiously insane are naturally of angry and violent dispositions, in the prime of youth, and of a plethoric constitution, and tense fibre.

Furious signs of violent disposition.

2d. They lose all their natural delicacy of manners, and become furious, ungovernable, and are particularly affected by pride, anger, hatred, and revenge, and very often intemperate lust.

Subject to passions.

3d. They refuse their food, and yet preserve their strength; they scarcely ever sleep, are continually shifting their ideas from one thing to another; bear

Refusal of food.

G   the

the cold with incredible patience, and are not easily affected by medicines.

Peculiar look.

4th. They have a peculiar look with their eyes, descriptive of violent anger mixed with a glariness like that of drunken persons, their eye-lids are constantly vibrating, and their hands, and sometimes the whole body, they keep in motion.

Melancholic.

Melancholy persons are,

Phlegmatic.

1st. Naturally dull, slowly learning, and easily forgetting, and are sad and melancholy, of a phlegmatic temperament, and relaxed fibre.

Fearful, &c.

2d. When the disorder seizes them they become abject, fearful, fond of solitude, prone to anger, changeable in their opinions and desires, but fixing their attention upon a single object.

Constricted in bowels, &c.

3d. The belly is constipated, the urine is made in small quantities; the abdomen is distended with wind; a sharp acrid matter is discharged by vomiting; the pulse moves very slowly; the

the aliment is devoured with greediness; the imagination is perverted so, as that they are persuaded that they are made of glass, china, &c. and lastly, and worst of all, they are induced to put a period to their existence.

4th. Their eyes have a dull, heavy, and stupid look; they seldom move, but continue in one posture a very long time.

Aspect dull.

CHAP.

CHAP. VIII.

OF IMPOSTORS.

Various
causes of
impositi-
on,
THERE are various causes which induce men to feign disorders to which the
human body is subject, and with such
fictions to impose often upon a court
of judicature, or at least a civil magistrate. To this they are induced from
fear, from bashfulness, or from lucre.
Should they be submitted to a physician
upon such an occasion, he can only
judge from the symptoms of the disease, and determine by their presence
and absence. But there are many
cases where artful people, by a speci-
ous tale, and by feigning disorders,
where much is to be known from their
own confession, may cause a good deal
of difficulty to discover the truth. Let
him

him then attend to the following circumstances.

1st. All the phœnomena which evi- Physician
should
consider
the phœ-
nomena.
ently appear in the subject at the time
of examination, together with such as
may be related by the sick person, or
the standers by, are to be carefully and
maturely weighed.

2d. An account is to be taken of the Take ac-
count of
natural
appear-
ances.
urine, age, pulse, hereditary disposi-
tion, way of living, condition of the
person, and the disorders to which he
has been subject.

3d. The questions which are to be Confound
the sub-
ject.
put to the sick person, or the by-
standers, are to be so framed as to con-
found them.

4th. The pretended sick person is Frequent-
ly visited.
to be visited frequently, and when he
least expects it.

5th. Enquiry is to be made whether Enquire
into
causes.
such causes as generally produce the
feigned disease have previously pre-
sented themselves.

G 3   There

Diseases feigned.

There are many diseases which may be feigned, particularly by a person who has before suffered from them, and especially if they be devoid of fever, and depend upon his own relation; yet there are but a few which are generally objects of imposition. These are epilepsy, melancholy, foolishness, possession by evil spirits, and fascinations.

Epilepsy.

1. A feigned epilepsy may be known from a real one,

1st. When the sick person does not fall to the ground very suddenly.

2d. When the face is not livid, nor the lips pale, nor is there any change made in the colour and real form of the face.

3d. When the patient is soon roused by sternutatories, or burning coals applied to the hands.

4th. When the nails do not appear livid.

5th.

5th. When the pulse is not altered.

6th. When at the end of the paroxysm the patient does not fall into a profound sleep.

7th. When he does not complain of a dullness of sensation, forgetfulness, a swimming of the head, great weakness, and thirst.

II. A melancholy that is feigned may be known by the absence of those symptoms mentioned in the last chapter. *Melancholy.*

III. We may conclude that foolishness is fictitious, when the person at any time appears rational : for persons afflicted in this manner are not furious as madmen, nor thoughtful as the melancholy, but speak confusedly, neglect themselves, and sing and talk like children. *Foolishness.*

IV. Possessions by evil spirits, as they constitute no real disorder, can *Possessions.*

never

never be feigned; the pretences therefore of such persons will not be detected by physicians.

Fascinations.

V. The same may be said of incantations, fascinations, &c.

CHAP. IX.

ON THE MEANS OF PRESERVING THE PUBLIC HEALTH.

THE general health of the public, which is of so much consequence, especially in large towns, calls loudly for the attention of the magistrate, who should exert every nerve to preserve and support it. This is best done by frequently consulting physicians of the first eminence, concerning the proper means to be embraced; and it would be highly useful if they were to be vested with proper authorities, and put in practice any scheme of this sort which they might think advantageous to the general service.

An object of consideration.

How best executed.

The health of the community seems in the best way of being preserved; when the following particulars are observed;

G 5.

observed; and it is no small matter to see them regularly put in execution.

1st. When every thing which may tend to injure the public health is properly prevented or averted.

2d. When care is taken that the sick have every assistance to remove the disease with which they are afflicted, or at least to mitigate its rage.

3d. When contagious and epidemical disorders. are guarded. against, and the spread of them, when they do prevail, prevented.

By averting the causes of disease.

I. The causes which are injurious to the health of the community may be averted,

By purifying the air.

1st. By preserving the air, as much as possible, from the effects of putrefaction, which must be done by. removing all kinds of putrid bodies, both animal and vegetable; for vegetables in this corrupt state are more offensive, or at least as much so, and consequently equally pernicious with animals.

animals. The lay-stalls of butchers
should always be situated at the extremities of towns, and large cess-pools
should be made, covered with earth,
to receive the blood and offal meat.
Buthers likewise should be punished
for keeping their meat till it be too
stale for use. It is not only improper
upon account of the smell, but poor
people, by reason of the reduced price,
are induced to purchase it, and thus
contribute to unwholesome diseases.

The water also of towns should be
carried off, and not suffered to stagnate in the streets. It is generally putrid in itself, but much more so when
it becomes a receptacle for all kinds of
filth. Hence we see that most towns
which are not accommodated with
common sewers, are very unhealthy.
The last thing to be considered under
this head are the burying grounds,
which should always be removed to
some distance from a town.

By wholesome provisions. 2d. The next means for removing the causes of injuries to towns, &c. is, by taking care that the corn be not of an unwholesome and putrid nature; that the flesh of animals be not diseased; that the fruits be properly ripened; that the wine be not poisoned, nor the beer foul and vapid; and that all vegetables of a deleterious quality, be not admitted to be sold.

By good water. 3d. By taking care that the water which is drank be tolerably pure, or free from any mineral substances, which may be prejudicial to health. This is not always easily ascertained, and will require a chemical analysis.

By regulating the use of spirits. 4th. By regulating the use of the still, and taking care that too much fermented liquors be not prepared.

By quantity of food. 5th. By providing a sufficient quantity of wholesome food for the use of the poor.

Suppressing stews. 6th. By suppressing the common stews, or at least regulating them in such

such a manner, as that the disorders
now peculiar to such places, and the
common effects of riot and drunkenness, be as much as possible, prevented.
In a moral light, no vice can be tole-
rated by the civil power; but in a physical view, we should certainly prevent
many of the deleterious effects of the
venereal disease, if not in time eradi-
cate it, by having the brothels under
the eye of the magistrate, who could
appoint inspectors under a licence,
who should regularly make their re-
port, and confine the subjects of it in
some well regulated hospital. If any
way then could be thought of, which
should avoid the encouragement of
vice, and yet admit of such an inspection, it would no doubt be of very great
benefit to society.

7th. By insane persons being pro-
perly confined and provided for. *Confining the insane.*

8th. By destroying mad animals;
and *Destroying mad animals.*

and when such are roving about, taking care that others are not suffered to go loose ; but confining them in yards, or other places within walls, &c. I do not think it proper to tie them up, as by their uneasiness and watchfulness, they may bring on them the disorders we would wish to prevent.

Suppressing quacks

9th. By suppressing as much as possible all mountebanks and quacks, and other pretenders to the practice of physic. No one can tell how much they injure society, by violent medicines, the effects of which they do not see; they may introduce some fatal disease, and by inefficacious ones they prevent the effects of those which are proper.

Preventing irregular practitioners.

10th. By preventing apothecaries, midwives, &c. from practice, unless properly recommended.

Preserving foundlings.

11th. By taking care that foundling infants, or others who may be deserted

serted by their parents, be taken care
of, and educated at the public expence.

12th. By preventing any persons
from selling drugs who are not bred to
the business of an apothecary or drug-
gist, or do not understand the nature
of medicines.

Regulating the sale of drugs,

13th. By regulating the shops of
those who sell drugs, so that the more
active medicines, such as vomits and
purges, emmenagogues, and the mineral acid spirits, be not promiscu-
ously arranged with the rest, but be
kept in some private drawers, or in an
inner room, to which no one should
have access but the master. At the
same time, particular care should be
taken of the labels, so that they make
distinct marks, &c.

And shops.

14th. That it be enjoined midwives and surgeons to call to their
assistance the most able physicians, in
cases of danger; and that for this purpose, physicians accommodate their
fees

Promoting consulta- tions.

fees to the abilities of the patient, so that all may receive the benefit of their advice.

Cæsarean operation. 15th. By midwives preserving the live child by a dissection, should the mother unfortunately die during the pains of labour.

Preventing diseases of cattle. 16th. By guarding against the contagious disorders which often arise among the horned and other cattle.

Diseases are removed: II. The best care is taken that the diseases of the sick be as speedily as possible removed,

By providing proper physicians. 1st. When physicians of great knowledge and the most liberal education are provided to order medicines, and illiterate and immoral men be not suffered to obtrude themselves on the public.

Public hospitals. 2d. When public hospitals are established, and so conducted as to accommodate all the sick poor who may offer:

3d.

3d. When surgeons and apothecaries, and midwives who are skilful in this business, are constituted by the public to execute their part of the business, which they undertake with carefulness and assiduity.

4th. When the apothecaries' shops are occasionally visited by the physicians, to see that their drugs are of the best quality, and provided in sufficient quantity for the exigencies of the sick : that their bottles and other vessels be preserved clean, and fit to contain the ingredients deposited in them : that the medicines be preserved in a proper place to preserve them from injury, and that the shopmen or apprentices be industrious, sober, and fitted for their business.

III. The next thing to be attended to is, by what means contagious and epidemic diseases are to be prevented and removed. These are of two kinds, what is called the plague, or any other disease

disease of the same nature, though less deleterious.

I. The plague is a disease of so alarming a nature, that every precaution should be taken by magistrates to prevent its access.

The following seem to comprehend the principal regulations necessary to be observed.

1st. The purification of the air is to be studied, and every thing put in execution that can promote this end. Some have proposed, for this purpose, the explosion of great guns, the lighting up of fires, &c. These can only have effect in rarefying the air, as heat is found to contribute to promote this disease, as described by Doctor Mead. The church bells, for the same purpose, are frequently to be rung; and the greatest cleanliness in the streets, and all public places, is to be observed. Besides this, sulphur and pitch, &c. may be burnt in the

open

open places, and vinegar may be evaporated in the chambers and insides of houses, as well as the fumigation of juniper and other woods be kept up.

2d. Lines are to be formed, which are not to be transgressed by the infected, nor by the healthy; at the same time, proper houses are to be allotted for those who are taken down in the disease, and others for the healthy part of the family, where the disorder prevails. Forming lines.

3d. All commerce with countries, where the disease is prevalent, is to be avoided; nay some punishment should be inflicted on those who transgress this rule. It is an object of too much consequence to be neglected, the lives of so many thousands depending on it. Commerce forbidden.

4th. Vessels which come from such countries are to be driven from the harbour where they attempt to enter, and be obliged to unlade their goods, and properly ventilate them in some. Vessels not to enter harbour.

uninhabited

uninhabited island. I do not think the usual manner in which quarantines are performed by ships in harbour, are by any means adequate to the purpose. Were the plague really on board any such ships, forty or sixty days, no nor any time would be sufficient to prevent the disease, unless the goods were properly ventilated; bale goods being known to preserve the infection for many years: but, besides this, it is impossible to keep the superior officers of a ship from leaving it, and flying to their domestic mansions, to repose themselves after a long and tedious voyage. The only remedy is, to appoint a place for unlading and ventilating.

Appropria-
ting physi-
cians, &c.

5th. Physicians and surgeons, and ministers, are to be appropriated to visit the sick in the plague, and no others, lest the infection may be conveyed by them to sound persons. The same rule is to be observed with regard to midwives.

6th.

137

6th. Hospitals are to be provided for Providing hospitals.
the poor who may be sick of this dis-
ease, but every connection between
them and their friends should be prevented.

7th. The dead bodies are to be Buryin the bod
buried as soon as possible; and here
a suspension should be made of the law
against burying in any thing but woollen: nay that should be forbidden, as
it is a powerful retainer of infection.
Linen here should be preferred.

8th. Every thing which is capable Cloaths, &c. burying.
of retaining infection, as the cloaths
of the deceased, and the furniture of
the room, should be buried. This is
preferable to burning. Those things
which retain infection the most, are,
all sorts of woollen cloths, silks, cot-
tons, linens, the skins of animals, hemp
and flax, &c.

8th. The food of those who are not Regulating food of healthy.
infected at such a time, should be prin-
cipally of vegetables, and of those
which

which contain the acid salt pretty
strongly, together with all sorts of
fruits. The chewing and smoaking of
tobacco may also be recommended.
But the best preservative is a mind
free from care and anxiety.

Similar
disease.
II. In diseases which are less
extensive than the plague, but still
highly infectious, and sometimes dangerous, the following should be re-
garded.

1st. Physicians should study the
nature of these remedies appropriated
to them, and consider with care what
are most likely to remove them.

2d. The poor are to be moved into
hospitals, and placed in wards by
themselves.

3d. The sick, even in private fami-
lies, should be separated from those
who are healthy.

4th. The healthy should live upon
a spare diet, nor indulge to excess either in wine or venereal pleasures; the
air

air they breathe should, if possible, be purified.

5th. Chewing tobacco and other herbs, and other preservatory medicines should be used.

6th. Flowers growing in pots should be introduced into sick rooms, as well as aromatic herbs. This should be done likewise in courts of judicature, where it is feared that the gaol distemper prevails.

FINIS.

Printed by Smith & Davy, Queen Street, Seven Dials.